Natural Therapies for Symptoms of Parkinsons Disease is an extraction of one chapter from Road to Recovery from Parkinsons Disease by Robert Rodgers, Ph.D. (2013).

I0413293

TABLE OF CONTENTS

Natural Therapies for Parkinson's Symptoms

Natural Therapies for Parkinson's Symptoms

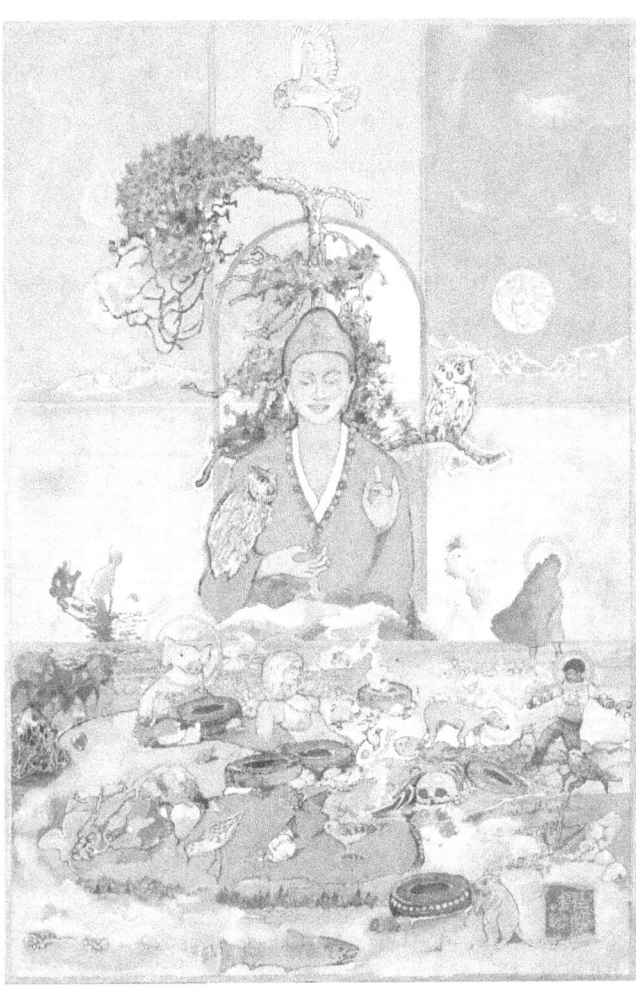

Medicine Buddha (2003) Michael Sawyer

DYSKINESIA

Dyskinesia is a jerky, dance-like movement of the arms and/or head which typically occurs after several years of treatment with L-DOPA or levodopa. The surgical procedure known as deep Brain Stimulation (DBP) is sometimes recommended when the "on" periods of the medications begin to shorten.

There is an alternative to DBS that also increases the length of time that levodopa is effective (the "on" periods). Citicoline is a nutrient for brain health that has been shown to be effective in reducing the dose of levodopa that is needed by as much as 30-50%. Citicoline is a natural substance derived from soy and egg yolks that is available as an over-the-counter supplement in health food stores. It has few side effects and costs less than most prescription medications. The dosage of levodopa usually has to be adjusted when Citicoline is taken, so it is important to

Natural Therapies for Parkinson's Symptoms

consult with your doctor if you want to pursue this alternative. Find more information about this alternative in *Natural Therapies for Parkinsons Disease*.

Pamela Quinn has observed that Michael J Fox is brilliant in how he moves his body. He is continually shifting his body in all directions as he talks. He follows the way his body wants to move rather than resist and face the possibility of freezing up.

Pamela Quinn has also found that applying pressure can be helpful. For example, if you have a lot of dyskinesia or tremor in your head, ask a friend to press on the two sides of your head with their hands. If they apply pressure with a little force, your body will relax and your head tremor will subside.

TREMORS

A wide variety of supplements have been suggested to me for the treatment of tremors. One in particular stands at the top of the list magnesium. Magnesium helps to reduce tremors and facilitates natural detoxing of heavy metals and other harmful substances. I rub magnesium lotion on my body and spray oil under my arm pits every day from Ancient Minerals: www.ancient-minerals.com

The herb Ashwagandha has been identified in research as a useful remedy for tremors, freezing and muscle pain. Rosemary tea is a natural treatment that facilitates the brain body communication, easing mobility challenge which can arise from time to time.

Professor Dancer Pamela Quinn uses some counter intuitive approaches to control her own tremor:

> I take charge of the tremor. I shake the tremor. I don't let the tremor shake me. I do it. That way I am manipulating it. I am taking control of it. There is this sort of psychological benefit as well as a physical one.
>
> Then, when I release my arm the muscles are relaxed for a bit. The tremor won't go away totally. It will come back. Then I do that again.
>
> If I am in a social situation where I do not want to look like a crazy person shaking my body around - I will put my hand under my leg. When my tremor starts up I shift position. I will put my hand on my hip or behind my back. If my tremor starts up I will shift it again. I will even sit on my hands.
>
> As soon as my body enters a physical behavior that I don't want I interrupt it and I shift to another mode. That is a way of saying
>
> "No. I am not going there."

Natural Therapies for Parkinson's Symptoms

People report that use of herbs such as Barley Malt Extract, Rhodiola Rosea Mucuna and Fava Beans offer them relief from tremors. Whether any of these herbs can actually help you depends on the level of dopamine in your body and whether or not the dopamine that is present is actually being absorbed. Herbs are just as much a medicine as Sinemet. It is important to consult with your doctor when supplementing prescription medicines with herbs.

LACK OF ARM SWING

For some people, one or both arms stop swinging when they walk. Ask yourself the question – why does one of my arms (or both arms) not swing like they used to? Your body is always protecting you in one way or another. If you force your arm to swing, you may experience freezing or tremoring on an opposite leg.

Experiment on yourself. What happens when you swing your arm? What other parts of your body are affected? Instead of viewing the lack of arm swing as an impediment, it may well be the case that this is your body's way of protecting you against a fall or freezing.

Professor Matt Ford, Ph.D. explains that you get better at what you practice. If you practice swinging your arms, you will eventually have a better arm swing. If you try and think about coordinating your arm swing with you steps, you will probably succeed in the short run. No one however can sustain their focus on the mechanics of walking. It is an automatic process that cannot be mechanized.

Focus helps in the short run but in the long run it flops. What is the alternative? Matt Ford has the answer: Walk to the beat of music you like to hear. The arm swing becomes more natural when it is matched to rhythmic beats.

What music is best? Music you like to hear and music that has a strong beat. Professor Ford suggests that everyone listen to music as often as possible. It is an eloquent, simple solution to a perplexing problem.

Professional Dancer Pamela Quinn also offers a simple, yet effective solution to this problem which she explained during my radio show with her:

> *"If you take a grocery bag that has some food in it or anything weighted and you swing that from front to back - that will help get that arm moving."*

FROZEN SHOULDER

Angela Wensley has found that intramuscular stimulation (IMS) has been a very effective therapy that lengthens the muscles that have shortened due to misuse. Here is her explanation of IMS:

Natural Therapies for Parkinson's Symptoms

"IMS involves needling as in acupuncture but the needles are applied to the tendons instead of to fictional meridians. The benefits of IMS are immediate and last for at least several days. I see my physiotherapist weekly."

Johan Boswinkel finds that the root cause of frozen shoulder is a digestive system that is malfunctioning. Work on getting your digestion back on line and the frozen shoulder problem will resolve.

FOOT DRAGGING

As a soccer Mom, Pamela Quinn invented a solution to her foot dragging which works beautifully for her. She puts a soccer ball inside a plastic grocery bag and proceeds to kick the ball with her lazy leg. After helping the body to renew the neural pathways that are required to wake up a lazy leg, she puts the soccer ball aside and pretends she is kicking it. Try it if foot dragging is a problem. It works.

Howard Shifke had difficulty stepping onto the first step of his stairs. Initially, he held onto the stair rail and used his upper body strength to walk up the stairs. This distorted his posture and twisted his body. He then switched to a more calculated and docile approach. He held onto the rail and placed one foot on the next step. Then he placed his second foot on the same step. It took longer to walk up the stairs, but he did so without exerting upper body muscles or distorting his torso.

Howard found that less was more. Mobility challenges will totally exhaust you by the end of the day because muscles are continuously been challenged and flexed. Howard found a much better approach was to move slower and more mindfully. He never pushed his physical limits. He always walks slower than necessary. This way he was able to maintain a reserve of energy when it was most needed. Howard is symptom free today.

FALLS

Professional Dancer Pamela Quinn has a unique appreciation for the mechanics of movement. Here is her recommendation offered during my radio show for prevention of falls:

It is important to lead with your feet - to lead with your heels in particular as a way of preventing yourself from falling or tripping. In Parkinsons you tend to lead with your torso.

Sometimes I have people pretend they are on a fashion runway because it puts their chest up and their shoulders back and it makes their feet lead. If you are going backwards it is also very important for your feet to lead. The tendency with going backwards is for your upper back to go back. That can lead to a backward fall. You want

6

to crouch forward and make your feet go back. Your body should always follow where your feet go.

FREEZING

Here are professional dancer Pamela Quinn's secrets to avoid freezing:

"There are different ways to take detours in your neurological pathways. One way is to take giant steps. Or, you are going to walk quietly. You can become a Marx Brother and bend your knees and take those big low steps. Anything that will take you out of your Parkinson's movement pattern and shift you into a different reality can be something that breaks through your problem and allows you to get going.

When I cross the street I either step over those white lines or on each one. I give myself a task which is related to visual cuing. Sometimes I use the visual cuing and the oral cuing together. If I have my IPOD, I sync up to music. I have all kinds of categories of music - so I am in a rhythm with my gait as I step over the cracks in the sidewalk.

One thing I did for years in walking is to place myself behind someone - not too close behind - and I sync my walk with theirs. I would take their rhythm. I would take their gait. It would help even out my gait. They would turn and I would find someone else to follow.

Just the other day there was a person walking with a pair of heels. I could hear: Click. Click. Click. Click. So, I put my walk right into her rhythm of the sound of her feet. Both visual and oral cues have helped me tremendously in working my body to move in as normal a way as possible."

Pamela also suggests that you attach masking tape on your hallway or floor. Increase the distance between each tape marker. The challenge is to step over the tape (not on the tape) as you walk. Your stride will increase because the distance between the tape markers increases. This will open up your stride and improve your gait.

Physical Therapist Kevin Lockette offers the following suggestion to address the perplexing challenge of freezing.

"I just read an attentional focus study that addressed teaching people strategies on how to move. There are basically two different ways to teach. They examined focusing on internal cues like your own legs or external cues which is something away from your body. In these studies, the external cues help people unfreeze and help people get out of it. For instance a lot of predictors that will trigger freezing are:

- *elevators*

- *escalators*

- *turning corners*

I train the people so that when they encounter those circumstances they can avoid freezing. One strategy is always to focus away from their body. For instance, if we are having a problem with freezing in an elevator and there is a lot going on –

- *You have anxiety.*

- *There are multiple elevators.*

- *Which one is going to open first?*

- *Can I get there before it shuts?*

- *How many people will be on the elevator?*

- *How long does it take for the elevator door to shut?*

All of these things can increase symptoms for people. If people have these strategies, the anxiety goes down. The external cuing is basically looking at the destination of where you want to go.

I always have people look past the threshold. If a threshold is the trigger of your freezing, I will have them focus not on their feet, not even on the threshold, but past the threshold – where they want to go on that elevator. I have them focus right on that spot and walk toward it. A lot of times it can be effective and they will not freeze.

A lot of times when people freeze both your legs are loaded. You are literally frozen. If you do not have a strategy you may try to move with both your legs loaded (which can throw you off balance) and sometimes fall. I will teach people to stop and try to take control. Basically, cautiously move.

One of the staples that I teach everybody is what I call the poor man's hula where if you are frozen, your weight shifts back and forth left to right like you are swinging your hips like a hula dancer. You can do this very subtly. You can do this maneuver in 3-5 seconds. You just shift to one side, shift to the other and then purposely take the first step towards a target away from your body. It pretty much works a majority of the time. Those types of strategies are helpful.

Natural Therapies for Parkinson's Symptoms

The whole idea is by shifting your weight you are going to off load the weight and now you can pick it up. The benefit of swaying is that now you are moving cautiously. Cautious movement will help get you out of freezing. The problem with freezing is that people don't have the strategies. They are operating on this automatic pilot that is not working. You turn off the automatic pilot especially during the freezing periods and then move consciously.

In most circumstances you can move out of it. The side to side weight shifting – the poor man's hula – forces you to turn off the faulty automatic pilot. You are grounding the steering wheel and driving your body yourself. You teach yourself to do that. You consciously are thinking about your movement. The weight shifts to one side. This off loads that leg and you can pick it up. Again, my experience has been if you can focus on where you want to step it seems to work better."

Howard Shifke (http://www.fightingparkinsonsdrugfree.com) invented a different way of solving the challenge of freezing that he faced. During the initial diagnostic assessment, his neurologist asked him to put his left arm out. To Howard's surprise, his right leg began to tremor. A similar result occurred when he put his right arm out – his left side began to tremor. While everyone knows that the right brain controls the left side of the body and the left brain controls the right, Howard speculated that he could rewire his circuits to avoid setting off undesirable tremors and freezing. When he learned to control the right side of his body with his right brain and the left side with his left brain, all would be well.

For example, Howard noticed that his left hand sometimes froze when he drove. Since he was accustomed to holding the steering wheel with his left hand and pushing on the gas pedal with his right foot, these episodes were genuinely problematic. He figured out by analyzing the electrical impulses in his body that the source of freezing in his left hand was caused by his right foot (which of course was on the gas pedal).

What was his solution? He started putting his left hand under his left thigh (to prevent his habit of holding the steering wheel with his left hand). When he holds the steering wheel of his car with his right hand he experiences no freezing episodes in his arms or legs. By stimulating the right side of his brain to move the right side of his body and stimulating the left side of his brain to move the left side of his body, all movement challenges were eventually resolved.

SLEEP DISORDERS AND INSOMNIA

Do you have problems sleeping at night? John Coleman, ND who once had Parkinsons himself and now helps others in his role as a naturopath doctor offers the following suggestions.

Natural Therapies for Parkinson's Symptoms

"Now this is a difficult challenge for those of us with Parkinson's disease symptoms. A poor sleep pattern can result from pain, restlessness, a neurotransmitter imbalance between serotonin and melatonin, adrenal stimulation, lack of exercise or lack of fresh air."

"It seems weird sometimes because we can - in fact we often do - feel really tired to the point of exhaustion. Yet we go to bed and cannot go to sleep or if we go to sleep, we wake frequently."

"Some of the things that can help are meditation before bed - say 10 minutes. There are some really good CD's to help that if we need that. Some of them can be played softly in the bedroom or some can be listened to through stereo headphones."

"Magnesium powder taken after dinner sometimes helps settle restlessness so that we go to sleep easier. Homeopathic magnesium phosphate or some other homeopathic remedies like coffea or chamomilla can help you sleep. Herbal mixtures like Passionflower, Hops, Jamaica Dogwood can help."

"One of the important aspects of this is to not become worried or anxious about the lack of sleep because that then sets up a negative feedback pattern. Our sleep pattern becomes even worse."

"We need to move around during the day as much as we can, particularly if we can get outside, that is good. Keep physically active. We need to get as much fresh air as we can. Make sure we do some stretches before bed to relax our muscles."

"Often we will sit all evening and then get up and go to bed. Our muscles have gotten quite tight and short so we can't get comfortable. If we do some stretching, some Pilates stretching, or yoga stretching or simple stretching before bed, that will often help our muscles relax better."

"It is also really important not to just turn off the television and go to bed. Television stimulates bursts of neurotransmitters in our brain that sets up sort of a chattery situation. If we just switch off the television and go to bed our mind is still chattery. It is important to have 10 minutes or so of quiet time, after we have switched off the television, before we go to bed and go to sleep."

I also would like to respond to this question using my own experience as a guide. I have attended seminars where doctors give step by step instructions that are supposed to help you sleep. You have probably heard the same recommendations: Go to sleep at the same time every night, don't watch TV before you sleep, eat (or drink) ... etc.

Natural Therapies for Parkinson's Symptoms

Speaking for myself, I cannot do these things before I sleep. The routine is too rigid for me. My life is too unstructured. If you have a similar response, you might want to investigate any one of the six strategies I have listed below. Surely one will be the winning ticket for you if you have problems with your sleep routine.

Ear Plugs

It may sound silly, but many people are very sensitive to sounds. Spend a $1 at the dollar store. Buy some wax type ear plugs (like swimmers use). Put them in your ears before you sleep.

Exercise

When I exercise during the day, I am much more likely to get a good night's sleep. Sweat works wonders when it comes to rest.

White Noise

We turn on an air cleaner at night when we sleep. It is a soothing way to screen out extraneous noise that can put your hormonal system on alert. Noises that come from unknown places in the dark create fear in the body which is bound to keep you awake.

Darken the Bedroom

When we started closing the blinds in the bedroom at night, we discovered it is much easier to sleep. For years we looked out the windows at our beautiful view of the Puget Sound, but at the cost of restful sleep at night. Darkening the room promotes sound sleep.

Holosync

This is my personal favorite strategy for sleep, though it is the one recommendation that costs a little money. If I am ever unable to sleep, I pop on my holosync ear phones. I am out in two minutes.

Acupressure

Some people report that a brief acupressure treatment in the evening offers them a good night's sleep. Like acupuncture, acupressure activates meridians in the body using gentle pressure, but using your hands and fingers rather than needles. You can apply acupressure on yourself or ask your spouse to do it for you every evening. A few minutes can work miracles if you are having difficulty getting to sleep.

Protein

Kristen Allott, ND, (www.dynamicpaths.com) argues that the body needs protein to maintain the right balance of hormones that are conducive to a restful night's sleep. She recommends that anyone who is having sleep challenges eat a little protein just before going to bed. Give it a trial run. I predict you will be pleased with the result.

Natural Therapies for Parkinson's Symptoms

EYE PROBLEMS

Are you having issues with your eyes? Perhaps dry eyes. Perhaps double vision. Perhaps jittery eyes. Perhaps cloudy eyes.

My uncle Gordon Ward developed advanced cataracts at age 65. A former college president of Sheridan College and Wyoming State Legislator, Gordon loved to play tennis, read books and write about history. Cataracts made it so difficult for him to read that Gordon reluctantly decided to have cataract surgery, one eye at a time. There was no other good option in the 1990's.

Cataract surgery on Gordon's right eye healed beautifully. Surgery on the left eye was a miserable flop. Gordon developed double vision and for all practical purposes was blind. He could not read. He could no longer play tennis. It was all a horrible mess.

My Aunt Betty said that the stress of cataract surgery caused Gordon to begin experiencing the symptoms of Parkinson's. He was diagnosed shortly after his botched surgery. Had Gordon been able to see, I believe he would still be playing tennis today. He died in the spring of 2009. Only later did we discover that Gordon had hepatitis C, not Parkinson's.

As part of my work to identify natural remedies, I am excited to report that I found a natural antioxidant eye drop that reverses cataracts and addresses other eye problems caused by inflammation. Had this antioxidant therapy been available to Gordon he could have reversed his failing eyesight without resorting to cataract surgery. Obviously, cataract surgery is a viable option for many people, but for my Uncle Gordon it was a disaster.

The discovery of an antioxidant remedy originated with the work of a Russian medical biophysicist Mark Babizhayev, Ph.D who made the simple, but profound observation that people who had no eye problems had sufficient levels of N-Acetyl-Carnosine in their eyes. People with cataracts and other eye problems had insufficient levels of N-Acetyl-Carnosine in their eyes.

Dr. Babizhayev took his research to the next level ten years ago by formulating eye drops that contained N-Acetyl-Carnosine which he called Can-C. He then began doing research to see if this antioxidant eye therapy worked.

Studies confirmed his hypothesis. Add the Can-C eye drops to the eyes and the eyes are able to heal naturally. Cataracts were reversed in about 95% of the cases. The Can-C eye drops resolve eye problems because they reduce the inflammation that is aggravating the problem in the first place. Isn't that totally cool?

Natural Therapies for Parkinson's Symptoms

I also want to make the obvious observation that our eyes are physically located next to the part of the brain that is responsible for manufacturing dopamine. I am wondering if healing eye problems might have an indirect, but positive impact on Parkinson's symptoms in general. The jury is still out on that one, but you never know...

You can find more information about Can-C eye drops and Dr. Babizhayev's research by visiting: http://www.cataracts.parkinsonsrecovery.com

I have aired two radio shows on the antioxidant Can-C eye drop therapy - an interview with company representative Jennifer Jones from Innovative Vision Products on February 11, 2010 and an interview with both Jennifer Jones and Dr. Babizhayev that aired April 1, 2010.

CAN-C PLUS. When I interviewed Dr. Babizhayev, he could not stop talking about his recent revelation concerning a dietary supplement that he formulated which bolsters the anti-inflammatory effects of Can-C eye drops. People who have advanced cataracts need extra support to reverse them, so he formulated a full spectrum antioxidant supplement that contains carnosine and an array of other antioxidants. This particular supplement gives people with advanced cataracts the extra boost that is necessary to reverse their cataracts.

Apparently, Can-C Plus does much more than to help reverse cataracts and address other eye complications that are caused by inflammation. Dr. Babizhayev's recent research shows that the Can-C Plus nutritional supplement reverses the increased aging effects of chronic illnesses at the DNA level. How can this be?

Can-C Plus lengthens telomeres which become shorter with natural aging and the cellular damage caused by all chronic illness. A telomere is a region of repetitive DNA at the end of a chromosome which protects the end of the chromosome from deterioration. His findings show that shortening of telomeres is not just stopped. Rather, it is reversed when Can-C Plus is used as a supplement. That is, the telomeres become longer!

Don't get me wrong here. Dr. Babizhayev has not done any research with Parkinson's patients, though I encouraged him to launch such a study. He makes no claims about what Can-C Plus can do for the symptoms of Parkinson's. But, I wonder if the Can-C Plus supplement might also provide sustained relief from the neurological damage caused by Parkinson's. If you are taking the Can-C Plus supplement, please let me know about your experience so I can document it. Discover more information about Can-C Plus at: http://www.cataracts.parkinsonsrecovery.com

DEPRESSION

This is a truly challenging illness. The feeling seems to be trapped in a vice grip that will not let go. It seems as though nothing can pull you out of the depths of despair. Absent is the motivation to do anything of any substance. Present is the thought that nothing you do makes a difference. Clearly, hormonal imbalances are taking their toll.

Depression can be so deep and penetrating that it is nearly impossible to take any action to reverse it without help. Even making an appointment with a health care provider takes up too much energy. The negative thought form that emerges is:

"It won't make any difference anyway, so why bother?"

Depression is a place of despair where all you can think about is going to sleep so you are not haunted by the black void of nothingness and immobility. Have I described the sorry state of depression adequately?

THE VICIOUS CYCLE OF DESPAIR

A marked tendency for individuals who currently have a diagnosis of Parkinson's disease is withdrawal from doing activities that are enjoyable and fun. When you spend less time hanging out with friends and doing activities that have been intrinsically fulfilling in the past, you are bound to get depressed. As you pass up opportunities to feel good, depression creeps in your life. It may sit undetected until your friends begin saying to you:

"What is wrong? You look depressed."

The cycle is self fulfilling. You do less and less. You feel worse and worse every day. Hope spirals into a downward freefall. When feeling sad, most people put on hold doing any and all of the things that you most enjoyed doing in the past.

Psychologist Roseanne Dobkin, Ph.D., recommends that when you are depressed, act according to your goals rather than your feelings. No one feels like doing anything when they are depressed. If you act according to your feelings, rest assured you will become more depressed. We can normally be guided by our feelings, but in the case of depression, Roseanne Dobkin explains that feelings are an unreliable guide. Depression is anything but a normal state.

Focus on the goal of feeling better. Certain actions must be taken even though you do not feel like taking them. Once the depression lifts you can return to the practice of trusting your feelings.

HOW TO BEAT DEPRESSION WITHOUT MEDICATIONS

The most straightforward and simplest solution to reversing depression is to eat protein at two hour intervals throughout the day. I picked up this valuable suggestion from Kristen Allott, ND, a naturopath doctor who specializes in treatment depression and anxiety through the right nutrition. You may be thinking – "This is too simple to work" – or I should admit that was my first reaction. Part of me said that simple is better, so I gave it a whirl.

Natural Therapies for Parkinson's Symptoms

Her method works. Yea! In the past I tended to become fatigued and slightly depressed around 2:00 in the afternoon. Once I began eating protein more regularly, the spells of depression lifted. Benefits of eating protein are less fatigue, improved sleep, better energy, fewer bouts of hunger and more muscle mass.

What foods contain protein? Certainly meat and fish fits have high protein. So do many vegetarian foods such as tofu, tempeh, lentils, whole beans, garden burgers, quinea, millet, oats, brown rice soy milk, nuts, seeds, cottage cheese and yogurt. Dr. Allott suggests that you start the day with protein with a Lizard Brain Treat which consists of ¼ cup of fruit juice and ¼ cup of nuts. For more information on how to combat depression by eating protein more regularly, visit Kristen Allott's website: http://www.dynamicpaths.com

If you are taking medications, be sure and consult with your doctor about the appropriate quantity of protein for your diet. Eating too much protein can undermine the efficacy of certain prescription medications that are used to treat the symptoms of Parkinson's.

FRESH THINKING COMBINED WITH INVIGORATING ACTIVITY

What safe, natural and nonintrusive therapies provide relief from depression that is frequently associated with a diagnosis of Parkinson's disease? Here is a short list of Roseanne Dobkin's suggestions for ways to combat depression without having to resort to medications (which of course may be necessary for some people).

1. Exercise every day. Exercise boosts your mood and decreases stress. It doesn't matter what you do for exercise – just get your body moving.

2. Increase the time you spend every day engaging in activities that are meaningful, rewarding and pleasurable. Do you enjoy playing bridge? Then play bridge often. Do you enjoy playing tennis? Then play tennis often. Do you enjoy hanging out with friends at the local coffee shop? Then visit the coffee shop often.

Test out new activities you have never tried and see what happens. Ever bowled? Why not give it a whirl? Why not join a book club or investment club or women's group or men's group.

Professor Dobkin explained during my radio show August 19, 2010 that when people are depressed they overestimate the extent of their limitations. Acknowledge that tendency. Everyone does it. Put thoughts of limitation on hold. Experiment. If an activity is no fun - drop it and try something else. If you cannot make yourself act, hire a coach that will gently nudge you into taking action.

3. Acknowledge negative thoughts and then pause them. Are these thoughts really as true as you think? With depression, thoughts are influenced by emotions more so than logic. We automatically accept all of our thoughts as true when in fact they are flat out silly or dead wrong. When we become depressed, negative thoughts are seldom as true as we think they are. They are also rarely accurate. Replace negative thinking with a more balanced view.

4. Treat every challenge as a problem solving opportunity.

> *You can't go to the party because you cannot drive? There is a solution to this problem. Find it and go to the party.*

> *You don't want to go out to dinner because you are having difficulty holding a fork? There is a solution to this problem. Solve the problem. Go out to dinner. Have some fun.*

Become more flexible. Make fewer demands on yourself. Depression is not a normal state of affairs. Act accordingly.

Elizabeth, a guest on my radio show, offered a lucid explanation of how she was able to function so beautifully despite having been diagnosed with Parkinson's two decades ago. Her trick was to carefully plan out each day so there was enough time to accomplish everything without rushing or stressing. She learned how to pace herself and move through each moment of her day with the grace of an angel.

5. Finally, Professor Dobkin recommends that if you are depressed, find a method of relaxation that works for you. There are many options including visualization, progressive muscle relaxation, deep breathing, meditation, self-hypnosis and others. You probably already have a method that works for you. Use it on the spot when you are stressed.

Music

Professor Matt Ford, Ph.D. during my radio show on January 26, 2011 suggested that listening to music can provide welcome relief from sour moods. Play music around the house all the time as often as possible. Music helps you move with ease. Music helps with balance. Music has a powerful emotional impact. Music increases endorphins (which are the pain killers). Music enhances mood. You will move better, feel better and smile more often.

Depression can be very problematic if you happen to live in the northwest United States during winter time. What follows is my short list of strategies I have personally found to be useful for fighting off depression:

Natural Therapies for Parkinson's Symptoms

1. First, buy a seasonal affective disorder light. Use it every day. Drag yourself to the computer and order one online.

2. Second, purchase vitamin D3 and take it during the winter. Please note – this is D3, not a composite vitamin D supplement (which can include other forms of vitamin D).

3. Third, if there is sunlight, bask in it. You do not need to take D3 if you are able to get sufficient exposure to sunshine.

These are my simple suggestions because they work for me. You can pull these things off even in a state of deep depression. They will help pull you out of the darkness.

Take any or all of the steps above and you will see a gradual reawakening to the sweetness of life. If you are depressed and unable to act, get help. Asking for help is not a sign of weakness. It is a sign of strength and courage.

RIGIDITY

Physical Therapist Kevin Lockette from Hawaii suggests two exercises that will create more flexibility and reduce rigidity. He explains the problem resides in the lack of ability to rotate the hips freely. First, lie down on the floor or bed. Place both feet on the floor with your knees bent. Shift your legs to the left, then to the right. This simple exercise "oils" the hips joints.

Second, stand up. Pretend as though you are holding a golf club. Clasp your hands together and swing that imaginary golf club. When you do, you will feel the rotation in your hips. With each swing, the rotation becomes wider and easier. When the body is able to rotate at will, rigidity becomes less of a obstacle to effortless movement.

FACIAL RIGIDITY

Many people hold the mistaken belief that the source of the problem with facial rigidity – or social staring - is found in the facial muscles. As is the case with any localized issue in the body, the cause of the problem resides somewhere else. In the case of facial rigidity the problem is rooted in a spine which is rounded and hunched or a twisted pelvis. Body therapies help the problem of facial rigidity because they release the tension that is held and the misalignment that is found in the spine and pelvis.

Irene Pasternack explained in my radio show December 8, 2010 that when she helps you make little movements in your pelvis and shift how you balance on your sit bones, your sternum, chest and face are profoundly affected. It is easy to smile when the pelvis and spine are in alignment.

Natural Therapies for Parkinson's Symptoms

Feldenkrais™ removes the blockages and wakes up the neural pathways in the facial muscles. It is one therapy among others that offers the potential to reverse the embarrassing problem of facial rigidity that sends a misleading signal to others that you are uninterested in them and bored.

CONSTIPATION

Why should anyone be concerned about gut problems when "everyone" knows the challenge with Parkinsons involves a neural dysfunction? Function of the gut has a huge influence - I repeat huge - on the symptoms of Parkinsons. When the gut is working properly depression lifts, constipation is relieved and energy returns.

Let me be blunt. If your digestive system is not functioning properly, all of the money you spend on supplements and healthy food goes down the toilet.

The process is wicked. You spend money on supplements and healthy food. You pour the supplements and healthy food into your body each day like clockwork. The following day the supplements and healthy food from the day before come out the other end - unaltered. This happens over and over, day in and day out. Your body is not absorbing the nutrients.

There is a second reason to heal digestive issues such as constipation first if you have Parkinson's symptoms. People with neurological challenges are much more likely to have a store house of toxins such as heavy metals and pesticides that are trapped in cells throughout their body. If the digestive system is clogged up, these toxins cannot be eliminated.

To summarize:

You pour money down the toilet day in and day out.

1. *You do not feel any better.*

2. *You convince yourself it is impossible to feel better.*

3. *You stop doing the things that help you feel better.*

4. *End of story.*

The good news is that you can reverse this wicked cycle. Natural approaches for improving gut function are widely available. They fall into three categories.

1. *Increasing hydration in the body.*

2. *Maintaining a proper pH level in the stomach.*

Natural Therapies for Parkinson's Symptoms

3. Improving overall function of the bowel.

First let's consider the important role hydration which, as we age, becomes more and more problematic.

INCREASE HYDRATION IN THE BODY

If the body is not hydrated adequately, waste begins to accumulate in the cells. This is the underlying reason why many people feel sluggish and run out of energy by the afternoon. The solution is to hydrate your body.

John Coleman, ND recommends that people with Parkinsons take a homeopathic remedy for dehydration called the Aquas (www.aquas4life.com) This therapy involves taking a few drops of a unique combination of essential oils and Bach flower essences in the morning and the evening.

The mechanism in the body that signals thirst needs to be recalibrated as we age. I was totally unaware until last year that I had stopped drinking water. The tissues in my body had become chronically dehydrated. It is the type of problem that creeps up on you so slowly you do not even notice what is happening.

I have taken Aquas for about a year and have been amazed at their effectiveness. I now get thirsty when my body needs water. If I do not take the Aquas, I do not drink water because I am never thirsty. The Aquas have solved this problem for me. Discover more information about the Aquas homeopathic treatment by visiting http://www.aquas4life.com.

PH LEVELS

Everyone should maintain a pH level in the stomach of 2. The term "pH" is a measure of the acidity of a solution like a body fluid. The most acidic of liquids will have a pH as low as -5 (this is a negative five). The most alkaline of liquids have pH level of +14.

By way of comparison here is a sample of pH levels from selected foods: lemon juice pH = 2.4, coffee pH = 5.0, pure water pH = 7.0, tomato pH = 4.0, milk pH = 6.5.

A point of confusion for many people is to conclude that you need to eat more acidic foods in order to maintain the correct acidic content in your stomach. This is not true. Disease flourishes when the environment in the body is acidic.

A high proportion of the food you eat should contain a high alkaline content. Many doctors recommend that 60% of the foods should be alkaline. Others suggest 80% of the foods you eat should have a high alkaline content in cases of chronic conditions like Parkinsons.

Natural Therapies for Parkinson's Symptoms

Most people think of the acid-alkaline scale as linear: i.e., from 2 to 3 = 1 and from 2 to 4 = 2. It is not. Each individual pH unit is a factor of 10 more than the next higher or lower unit. An increase in pH from 2 to 3 represents a 10-fold change. An increase of 2 to 4 represents a one-hundred (10 × 10) fold change.

Shifting down from a pH level of 6 (which is very alkaline) to a pH level of 2 (which is more acidic) is thus not as easy as it might seem. Given the tricky nature of pH, is there any wonder that it is difficult to maintain the proper pH balance in the stomach?

The pH in the stomach needs to be low because acid is needed to break food down. Here is the key: If there is not sufficient acid in the stomach (i.e., the stomach is too alkaline), food does not break down. No. It crawls its way into your gut and - if you are squeamish do not read further - rots.

Please note that I said the pH level "in the stomach" should be around 2. The pH of other body fluids such as urine, saliva and blood vary considerably. For example, the pH of blood is 7.4. Secretions of the pancreas have a pH of 8.1.

In contrast, a fluid in the body that has a high acidic content in the body is plaque. Plaque's pH is low and will dissolve teeth if it is not removed.

How can you know if the pH level in your stomach is "2"? After all, having a pH lab test every day would be very expensive and time consuming.

There is an easy way to know. It costs nothing. It takes a second each day. Simply pay attention to the color of your bowel movements. OK. I know this is not exactly a sexy topic, but it is important to know.

If your poop is dark brown the pH level in your stomach is low enough. You are in good shape. If your poop is light brown, there is not enough hydrochloric acid in your system. That is to say, the pH level in your stomach is too high.

So if the color of the poop is too light corrective action is needed. What do you do? Take vitamin C and drink a lot of water.

Vitamin C is the body's antioxidant of choice. If we give our bodies enough vitamin C, our bodies are able to manufacture enough CoQ10.

There are many vitamin C products on the market, so be judicious in what you choose to purchase. I use a vitamin C product recommended by Randy Mentzer: Vital Mixed Ascorbates made by Pharmax which is loosely packed in a 9 ounce container. I mix it with water.

Natural Therapies for Parkinson's Symptoms

How much vitamin C should you take? Your body will tell you the answer. Just ask it. Muscle test yourself. You will need to take more and more vitamin C until your poop turns to a dark brown color.

Most people are unaware that our natural biology calls for large quantities of vitamin C. You may be shocked at how much is needed for your body to come back into balance.

IMPROVE OVERALL FUNCTION OF THE BOWELS

You are now well hydrated and your pH level is good to go. Now it is time to focus on getting your bowels moving. Everyone needs one good bowel movement every day. Two to three movements are ideal.

Herbs that can facilitate bowel function are gentian, chamomile, fennel and St Mary's thistle. Which herb (or herbs) will do the best job for you? I must sound like a broken record, but just ask your body. Muscle test yourself. Your body knows the answer.

Your body may be having difficulty digesting animal fats. I have received several reports from persons currently experiencing debilitating constipation challenges who switched to a vegetarian diet. Their constipation difficulties were resolved within weeks of the change in diet.

HOME REMEDY

John Coleman, ND recommends a homemade cocktail for people suffering from digestive challenges including constipation. He suggests you take this cocktail in the morning and evening 1/2 hour before meals. You make this special cocktail yourself.

THE RECIPE:

> *12 ounces pure water*
>
> *1/2 - 1 teaspoon vitamin C powder*
>
> *1/2 teaspoon magnesium*
>
> *1 ml (eyedropper) zinc liquid*
>
> *Aqua drops (1 drop AM in morning; 1 drop PM in evening)*
>
> *1 drop selenium*

Once you get your digestive system back on line, nutrients from the healthy food you eat will be distributed to the cells that desperately need to be nourished.

Natural Therapies for Parkinson's Symptoms

As always, check out my ideas to improve your gut function with your doctor before you decide to do anything. Always treat anything I say as information that needs to be discussed and evaluated with your medical doctor.

- May your constipation resolve with each passing day.

- May your energy rebound as your gut function improves.

- Your body and your pocketbook will thank you.

Memory Loss

People who have difficulty with their mental functioning often hold the belief the problem is centered in their brains. To be sure, this is the case for a very small proportion of persons. The root cause of memory problems for most people is much more likely to reside from a disruption in the healthy flora of their digestive system. The climate in their digestive track is too acidic. Good bacteria required for proper digestion vanish. Bad bacteria that disrupt the digestive process flourish. Without the presence of good bacteria in the digestive system, a person will see little benefit from eating organic, healthy food.

Find a doctor who is knowledgeable about the best probiotics to take (for your body) which can help your digestive system come back on line. When it does, celebrate a transformation in your cognitive functioning as your mind becomes sharp as a tack.

As another option, consider making your own probiotics. Sandor Katz has written a book titled Wild Fermentation which describes in detail how you can ferment foods in your kitchen and prepare your own probiotics. This is a fun, easy approach for helping your digestive system come back on line. You also get to prepare tasty fermented foods you love to eat.

Pain

Do you really want to rush into a strategy to eliminate pain? On the one hand – you probably have a knee jerk answer – Duh. There is another answer to this question which is not as popular as the first. From a holistic perspective, pain is a sign you are making progress on your road to recovery. Pain gives you valuable information about the cause of an imbalance in your body. If you are interested in healing the cause of the pain, it is best to hang out with it for a while rather than numbing it with medications.

Nutritional counselor Dorit offered a fascinating perspective on pain during my radio show on June 3, 2010.

Natural Therapies for Parkinson's Symptoms

"It is normal to have pain. I see pain as weakness leaving the body. I do not see pain as something to be covered up. The question is - how can we assist the pain in leaving in a smoother manner in a way that would help us to release the reason behind the pain if there is a reason to release it at all. Sometimes we need to just acknowledge and be there for our own growth."

In some cases, pain is the body's distraction from feeling unpleasant emotions like guilt, abandonment, rage, deceit, sorrow or grief. Instead of fixating on the pain, drop down just underneath the pain and ask yourself:

"What lies beneath this pain of mine?

You may be surprised at the answer. Once the wounds of unpleasant feelings are released, the physical pain disappears as fast as a parrot from a magician's hand during a magic show.

For reasons that may surprise you, meditation can be a powerful antidote to pain. Radio programs I offer on the subject of meditation are typically the least popular. I suspect many people believe little benefit can be derived from sitting in a silly position doing nothing. Norman Fischer explains why meditation can be extremely beneficial for anyone who experiences chronic pain.

To be sure, sometimes there is relief from the pain as a result of the meditation practice. I suppose it is not impossible depending on the condition there could be some significant change in the physical condition.... Generally ...it is a matter of:

- *How do we live with what we have?*

- *How do we manage it?*

- *If there is pain, how do we have some happiness and some relief even in the middle of some discomfort?*

The first head is - you have a pain. [With Parkinsons it may be pain in the muscles or joints] That is one head. Putting a head on top of your head is when you say:

"Oh, I hate this pain."

"Why won't it go away?"

"What did I ever do to deserve this?"

"How come nobody else has this pain?"

23

Natural Therapies for Parkinson's Symptoms

All of that actually becomes in many ways more painful, or at least as painful as the original pain. The idea is this. Can you accept and be present with the pain and take away that second head that you put on top. If you then just have the original head, life becomes much more bearable and sometimes quite beautiful.

How can you get immediate relief from pain when it is literally driving you up the wall? Michelle Mill's mother suffered from the persistent pain. She has chronic fatigue syndrome. It is not Parkinsons, but some of the symptoms overlap.

With a mother who was unable to find relief from any remedy that was prescribed by health care practitioners, Michelle took matters into her own hands. After months of trial and error experimentation she invented her own pain relief remedy that has proved incredibly successful. It has helped her mother and countless others.

Michelle told her own story of recovery on my radio show that aired September 10, 2009. You can also read additional information about her remedy by visiting www.iwokeupwell.com. She concocted the remedy by combining together every known analgesic including the natural form of aspirin which is derived from willow bark.

Call Michelle and talk with her about her remedy. Her phone number is on the contact page of her website. Michelle invented Willow Balm. She makes it herself. She helps people get immediate relief from their pain so they can attend to the underlying cause of it. It you are experiencing pain, this remedy is worth investigating further.

Will Willow Balm really help you get relief? Who knows? Everyone is different. But with free samples to try, why not experiment and see for yourself. Michelle is so proud of her natural product that she gives me free samples to give all Jump Start to Wellness participants.

RESTLESS LEG SYNDROME

Nutritional Counselor and Pharmacist Randy Mentzer offers the following recommendation for Restless Leg Syndrome.

> *"I lean toward trying natural products first. We find that magnesium glycinate works really well for restless leg syndrome. It is natural. It is a muscle relaxer."*

Music Medicine expert Suzanne Jonas, PhD, has developed an acoustic CD to treat restless leg syndrome by ear rather than mouth. Is that cool or what?

SALIVATION

Excessive salivation can certainly become one of the most troubling and at times embarrassing symptoms. Foot Whisperer Randy Eady suggests that you can always press on the acupressure points on the face that are directly linked to the function of salivation glands. He reports you can get relief for about 15 minutes (until the same points are pressed again). Press the jaw joint on each side of your face at the same time for 5-10 seconds. There is also a pressure point just below the ear hole on each side of the head.

Acupuncturists are of course the perfect resource in this regard. They can help you find the precise location of the acupressure points you need to press when relief is needed. Acupressure is a sweet self help therapy, something you can do for yourself whenever salivation becomes problematic.

STRESS

What can you do to get relief from stress? You are probably thinking to yourself –

> *I know what I can do to get relief from stress – but it costs me money. If I spend money – I will be even more stressed.*

Why not consider ways you can get relief from stress without spending a cent? Of course, it will still take a little time and effort on your part – but the outcome is well worth the effort. Learn how you can reduce your stress level (and see an immediate reduction in your own symptoms) by listening to my radio program interview with Keith Zang from the Moonglow Enlightenment Center that aired on January 28, 2010. Oh – I suppose I should clarify – it does not cost you a cent to listen to Keith's suggestions. You can always download any of my radio shows for free from the radio program website by visiting the show page. Scroll back to the February 28th show to hear my interview with Keith:

> http://www.blogtalkradio.com/parkinsons-recovery

Most people anticipate a happy retirement because the stressful demands of having a full time job can be terribly stressful. Some people count down the days until they will be free of the life style restrictions that are imposed by a 40 hour a week job.

Unfortunately, the expectation of a happy, stress free retirement is seldom realized. Most people are blindsided by the discovery that retirement itself is stressful. Here is the common sequence of events.

- *You just retired last month.*

- *You wake up in the morning.*

- *You confront the first decision of the day.*

- *You evaluate the possibilities: Walk the dog of take out the garbage.*

Natural Therapies for Parkinson's Symptoms

- *Then what?*

Such simple choices can be extremely stressed for a person who is used to making far more challenging and demanding decisions.

A passion is critical to managing stress successfully. If you have no goal for the day or week or month – if you have no reason to get out of bed in the morning - your hormones also have no reason to get out of their cozy beds either. It is hard to feel good when those hormones are always sleeping.

One successful approach for managing stress is to become more mindful each and every moment. Instead of anticipating the future (which creates stress) or regretting the past (which sustains past traumas), focusing on the present moment is a guaranteed way to reduce stress in your life. Becoming more mindful happens when you set your intention to live in the present. Becoming more mindful costs absolutely nothing!

Because I have such trust in mindfulness as a powerful, yet simple way to reduce stress, I created a Mindfulness Program which sends a challenge each week in the form of an email to become more mindful. Quite honestly, I developed this program because I was personally teaching myself to become more mindful. The Parkinsons Recovery Mindfulness Program costs a little money each week – the equivalent of one latte a week – so if paying out money for anything tends to create more stress in your life – the Mindfulness Program is clearly not the right solution for you.

Davis Phinney, the famous Tour de France cyclist who developed symptoms of Parkinsons, says that what has helped him is to take each moment as it comes. When you string the moments together, you wind up having a good day. If you spend your entire day thinking about what you cannot do, your chances of having a good day are slim. The mission of the Davis Phinney Foundation is to help people living with Parkinson's disease to live well today.

Most people believe that their minds activate stress hormones. Actually, the heart plays the leading role here. The mind is simply a "walk on" to the drama at hand. The opportunity to manage stress resides in the heart. When the heart relaxes, a signal is sent to the brain to relax. Open up your heart and watch stress in your life dissolve like a snowball in the sunshine. This therapy also costs nothing. Better yet, you pay nothing out and receive immense pleasure in return.

SWEATING

Here is what I see is happening with sweating. Remember I am a researcher, not a medical doctor, so be sure and consult with your doctor before taking any action.

Natural Therapies for Parkinson's Symptoms

Your body is sending you a strong signal. What is the message? I have a strong hunch that the lymph system is clogged. The system is simply not functional at present.

Why is it clogged? You may have an overabundance of toxins. Please do not be offended if sweating is one of your symptoms. First, my guess may be wrong. Second, everyone has this problem because we all live in a very toxic world.

When the body is attempting to do its work of eliminating toxins (which remember is one of its many jobs) and there are too many toxins for the body to eliminate through the kidneys, liver, bowels, etc) the body will use whatever means available to release the toxins. If the lymph system is clogged, the sweat glands are the alternative outlet.

Looked at from this perspective, sweating may be critical for the organs in your body to continue functioning. In other words, it is actually a good thing to sweat even though it is making you miserable.

What do you do about this? First, you can evaluate everything you put on your body, everything you eat and everything you touch. It is possible you are contaminating yourself in a most innocent way. It may be the shaving lotion you use. It may be your laundry soap. It may be the furniture you sit on has toxins.

Consider all possibilities. Eliminate any and all possible sources of toxins. Make it a project for the month. The source of the problem may lie in a most strange or obvious place, one that you never thought about before.

Second, you can purchase a small trampoline and jump on it for 4 or 5 minutes a day (unless balance is an issue for you). Jumping on a trampoline every day helps to clear out the toxins and clear your lymph system. I jump regularly. It is fun. It jiggles out the junk. The only way for the waste in your lymph to move is if you move. There is no internal pump that moves it out for you.

Third, you can contact a naturopath or medical doctor who can help you to detox gently. Or you can visit your health food store where there are usually people available who can answer your questions. There are many other natural options that can help you detox (infrared saunas, steam rooms, homeopathic treatments, etc.)

You also probably need to be especially careful to hydrate your body. You may have the thought that you do not want to drink water because it will make the sweating worse. Without adequate hydration, you cannot detox your body and your lymph system will remain clogged. I personally use a homeopathic treatment that was designed to address the problem of dehydration which works beautifully for me.

Natural Therapies for Parkinson's Symptoms

Herbal treatments can be helpful. Magnesium in the form of lotions or oils will facilitate the elimination of toxins in your body. A number of herbs will help clear out your lymph system and help you detox your body. I interviewed an amazing herbalist in Pioneers of Recovery, Andrew Bentley. Kate Tossey (www.katesherbs.com) has also been a guest on my radio show who is an amazing resource. Both herbalists are resources I would approach to get the best advice on herbs to try for detoxing my body. Consider essential oils as an option too. Aroma therapists like Jean Oswald, also a Pioneer of Recovery, are also wonderful resources.

Once the toxins have been cleared to a manageable state, your lymph system will begin to function normally and the symptom of sweating will hopefully subside.

SWALLOWING PROBLEMS

Why are swallowing difficulties so serious? The primary cause of death among people who have been diagnosed with Parkinsons Disease is pneumonia, a serious infection of the lungs. When food slides down the trachea (which leads to the lungs) rather than the esophagus (which leads to the stomach) the lungs are the recipient of food that create the conditions conducive to infection. Once food enters the lungs – there is no exit pathway other than back up the trachea by coughing.

You may not recognize you have a swallowing problem. Do tears flow from your eyes when you eat? Does your nose run when you eat? Do pills get stuck in your throat? Does your voice sound funny after you eat? If the answer is yes to any of these questions you probably have a swallowing problem.

I have problems swallowing pills, so I have recently become aware I have a swallowing problem. Roya Sayadi, Ph.D. and Joel Herskowitz, MD, authors of Swallow Safely, offer a recommendation which has helped me enormously. When I swallow it helps to tuck my head to my chest and turn my head to one side.

If you have a swallowing problem, make it a high priority to heal it. Sayadi and Herskowitz's Swallow Safely book is an excellent resource. I also suggest that you take the time to hear my radio show with them as my guests which aired on July 22, 2010.

Swallowing problems may be caused by TMJ disorders (jaw bone misalignments). If you have a swallowing problem consider having a dentist qualified to diagnose and treat TMJ problems do an evaluation.

INDEX

Natural Therapies for Parkinson's Symptoms

Natural Therapies for Parkinson's Symptoms

Natural Therapies for Parkinson's Symptoms